I am dedicating this Book To My former student Sabrina and many others to succeed in your career and learn to write great clinical notes. After reviewing many Dental Assistant Textbooks I have not come across even online search Dental Clinical Notes Cheats.

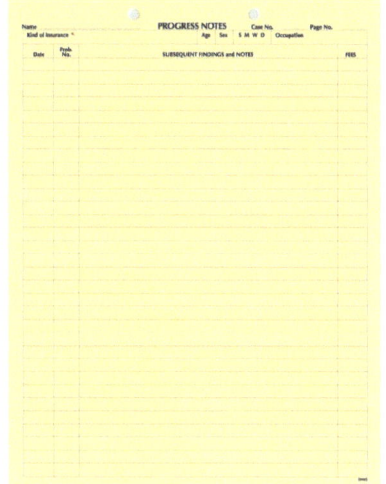

Progress Notes AKA Clinical Notes For Dental Professionals

Each Note may differ from the next depending on Anesthetic used, Treatment Performed including difficulties during procedure and Patient Information provide so be sure to adjust as needed and always ...always double check your notes. Think for you write because it is a legal documentation but just like you can get the rhythm down to explain Post Op instructions then you will do the same with clinical notes just changing it up as you go.

Quick tip: if you don't know your codes write the main one in each Procedure category for example if you know code for 1 surface Amalgam which is 2140

Clinical Notes

- Date 01/06/2018
  - Always put the date
- Exam Type
- X-Rays
- HH Review & Signed (each appointment should ask if any changes in Medical History and every 6 Months ask to have them sign and update HH = Health History Form.
- Always Put Your Initials if you type or write notes
- Always use Black Ink no Pencil!
- Always put one single line through it if a mistake do not white out nor delete or black marker
- Comprehensive Exam or Initial Exam Can Be Chosen Depending On DDS Request
- 2 BW's Write Code in if needed 0272 , or 4 BW's 0274 *(depending on Patient age and/or Dental Practice what they include in a Comprehensive Exam)*

- WNL which is an abbreviation for Within Normal Limits.
- NV=Next Visit
- *On Routing Slip Can Check off Treatment For Next Appointment or using Computer Software Click on required Page to enter Next Visit and time required so front knows how much to schedule and reminder each Dentist works at a different pace.*
- *P.O = Post Op Instructions*
- *More the Detail Notes The Better You are Covered in the Courts!*

On a separate sheet or on a note screen in the dental software can write a little something about patient to bring up the next appointment for example How is the Puppy doing you got last time. There is no way you can recall each patient story so write down Patient got new Puppy name Cotton. Never in the Clinical Notes you do not want your employer the Dentist reading what you wrote for example some might write Patient got a new puppy and peed on his shoes. Could you imagine that! I have first hand heard Dentist say they had to read some embarrassing notes to a court. Incase a procedure goes wrong Dentist would have to attend court.

Progress notes our a Patient's story line of their Oral Health

Examples

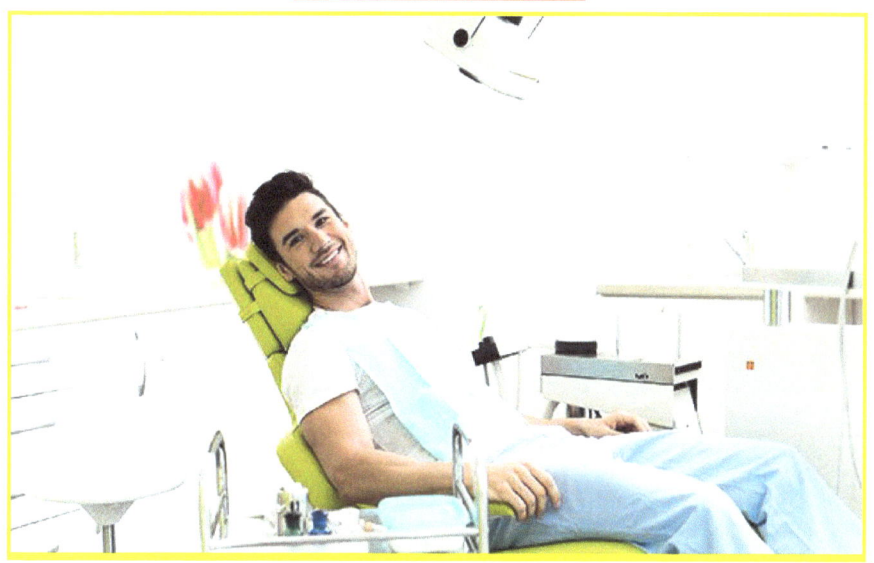

Initial exam

1/08/19 Health History Taken, HIPPA Form Sign, Initial Exam, 4 BW's, Panorex, Soft-Tissue WNL,Patient Photo & Intraoral Photos taken Patient Sign Refusal form for Continuing Care at this time due to toothache.

Patient came in with concern of Tooth #3 ,Took 1 PA which indicates recurrent decay under current crown which is over 5 years old and abscess is present. RX Prescribed Amoxicillin 300 mg 30 tabs Tiq 1 every 8 hours till gone, Patient did not want pain medicine due to former addiction.

NV: Endodontic Treatment #3
- Dr. RK , Asst./ T.B

Note: If Referring out Write Name of Dentist or Office

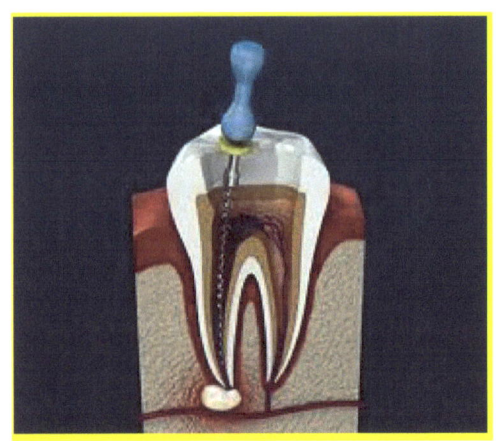

Endodontic Note Example

1/15/19   Pt completed Prescription as directed, Consent Form Sign for Endodontic Tx., B.P 120/ 80 ,Place Topical , Used 2 Carps of Lidocaine 1:100 , Patient did well with Anesthetic, Placed Rubber Dam

Tooth # 3 Open Canals Access and WL Files , DB 25 File at 21 mm , MB 30 File at 23 MM, took 2 WL PA's , Place Formocresol on a green sponge and Cavit in tooth and checked patient bite. Went over P.O Instructions with pt.

NV: Final Fill # 3

-Dr.RK, Asst. TB

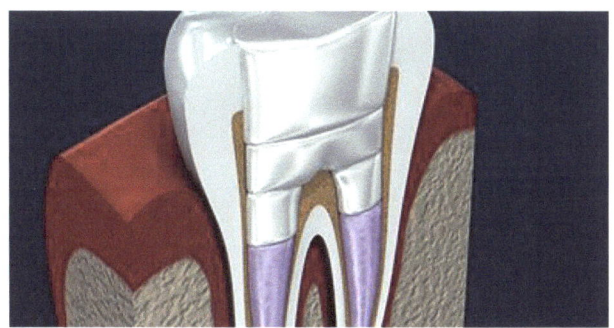

2nd Endodontic Appointment Note Example

1/21/19 B.P 123/80, Place Topical, Used 2 Carps of Lidocaine 1:100, Patient did well with Anesthetic. Placed Rubber Dam
Tooth #3 Removed Cavit and sponge, Used Gates Glidden to widen canals and removed remaining necrosis pulp. Irrigated with Peroxide followed by Hydrochlorite 50/50 mixed. Dry with paper points until clear, placed Tublisealer and 30 size Gutta Percha Points with 3 accessory points. Took Final Fill PA which shows canals are sealed. Patient tolerated procedure well.
NV: Crown Prep #3
-Dr.RK, Asst. TB

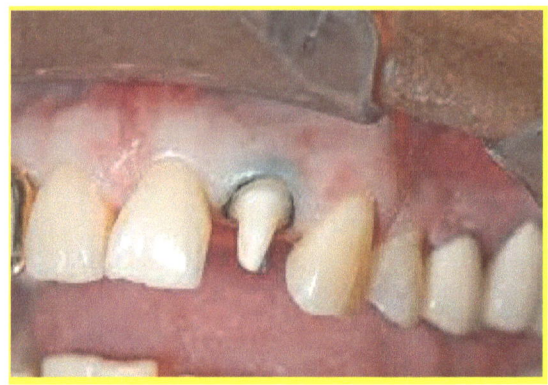

Crown Note Example

1/31/19 *Consent Form Sign for Crown on* Tooth #3 No Anesthetic Needed Patient had RCT , Placed Topical around Gingival tissue for comfort. Prep # 3 , placed 00 retraction cord, removed prior to taking final impression, Margins showed up well in impressions, Sent to Rogers Lab, Shade A3.5, Fabricated provisional coverage. Went over P.O Instructions with patient.
    NV: Seat Crown
    -Dr.RK, Asst. TB

    Note: Same way but change if using Cerec Machine to in office and no need for next visit to seat crown. If used a Post add that as well or Build Up.

    Note: If was referred out for Endodontic Tx, Write down what you removed from Endodontist office and have Letter Up on screen or Out for DDS

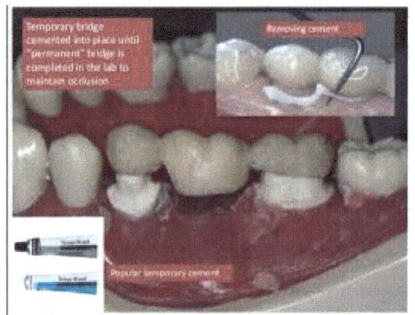

Temporary Crown Note

2/1/ 19 *Patient came in with Temporary crown off, Removed old cement remaining and check tooth all appears normal, Recement with Temp Bond and sent patient home with Temporary Cement packet in case it comes off again due to pt. Bruxism.*
-TB

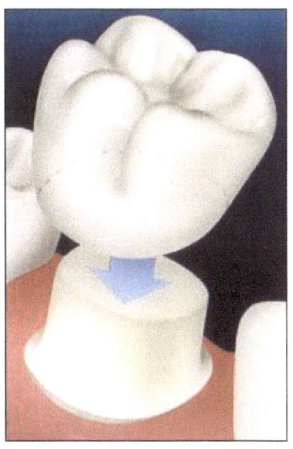

Seat Crown Appointment Notes

2/7/19 Patient came in with Temporary Crown Off , Check Shade with Patient to get approval and pt was happy with shade., No Anesthetic needed due to previous Endo tx., Clean tooth with Hemaseal Try on Crown and check contacts and bite, made necessary adjustments and seated crown with Ketac and removed any remaining cement. Went over P.O Instructions with patient.

    NV: Recall

    -Dr.RK, Asst. TB

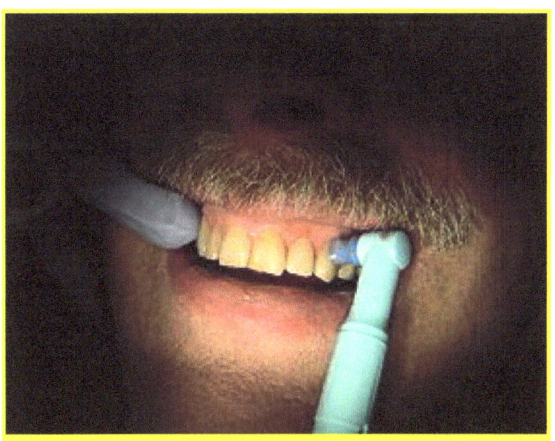

Recall AKA Recare and/or Prophy Note Example

2/15/2019 Perio Charting Completed and no pockets present or bleeding during probing.,Scale with Calculus present around tooth #24 L Surface, Took Intra oral Photo and went over OHI with Patient. Pt. Purchase Sonicare Toothbrush, Patient refused Fluoride and sign refusal.Concern over Health Factors in the news.

NV: Recare 6 Months

9/1/19 No Show No Call was confirmed LM with Patient To return our call
-TB
9/2/19 Patient called back and indicated was in a car accident on the way here and we dropped the broken appointment fee and reschedule appointments.
-TB

Note: Write in Red To Let Stand Out if Missed Appointment or Any Communication with Patient Over The Phone.

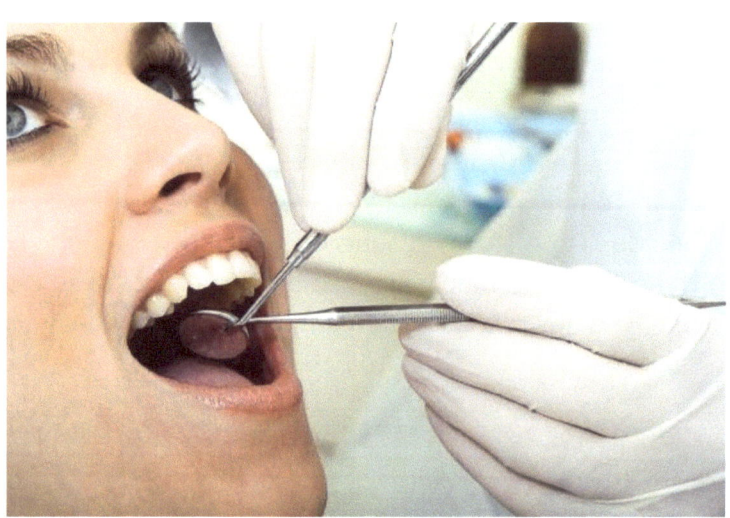

Limited Exam Note

11/1/19 HH Updated, Patient came in for Recall but had pain on LR side, Took PA could not find any indication for Abscess or Decay present. Did a Limit Exam and TMJ Exam and due to Bruxism Patient is to sore to stay open with Mouth Prop or with Breaks. Schedule Patient to come back for Impressions for Bruxism Splint for Night Time only. Advise patient to take OTC medicine as needed for pain. Use Ice for 20 minutes at a time if needed.
NV: Impressions For Splint
-Dr.RK, Asst. TB

Impressions Notes

11/2/19 Took upper and lower impressions and sent off to NDX for Splint for Bruxism, Also took patient bite registration and sent it to the lab.
NV: Seat Splint
-Dr.RK, Asst. TB

11/5/19 Seat Splint check patients bite with splint and made necessary adjustments, Went over care of New Appliance. Advised patient to bring in next Recall to clean it in our solution.
-Dr.RK, Asst. TB

11/6/19 P.O Call, Patient did well last night with appliance and headaches have stopped. Very pleased with it.
-Dr.RK, Asst. TB

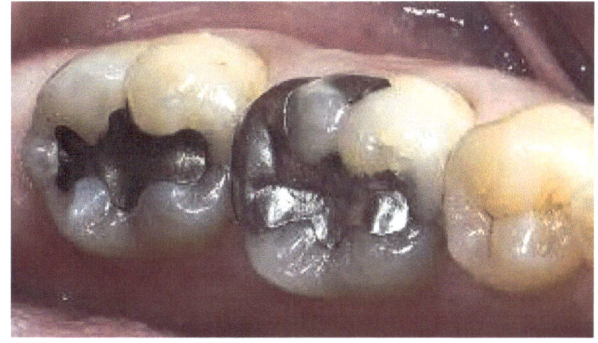

Amalgam Notes

1/1/20 No HH Changes, Emergency Exam, 1 PA # 30, No Pain associated with tooth not sensitive to hot, cold, or Sweets, #30 has an O Amalgam Restoration that came out due to recurrent decay present. Placed Topical, 1 Carpule of Lidocaine 1:100, Patient did well with Anesthetic, Removed remaining restoration, Placed Dycal liner, Used Matrix system and wedge for MO Amalgam. Check patient bite, During Tx #29 showed to have decay present on D surface, Patient did not want to complete due to pain in jaw due to staying open, Went over P.O Instructions.
NV: Composite #29
-Dr.RK, Asst. TB

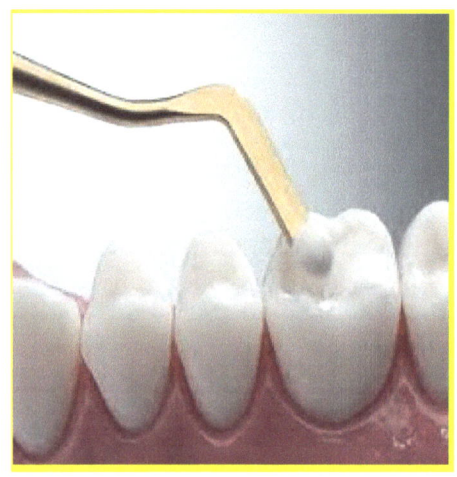

Composite Notes

1/3/20 Tooth #29 Placed Topical, 1 carp of Citanest 1:100 , Patient did well with Anesthetic, Removed decay present, Check with Sabel Seek all caries was removed, Placed Matrix System, Wedge, placed Etch, Bond, Shade A3.5 Composite, Light-Cured, Removed Matrix system and wedge, Check patient bite and was able to floss interproximally with no overhangs present. Went over P.O Instructions with Patient. Patient was pleased with shade and wanted to fix #8 due to old composite restoration has changed color.
Advise Patient if wanting Whitening will not be able to change the color of composite once done, Patient indicated she would like to have whitening prior to Restoration.
NV: Whitening Trays
-Dr.RK, Asst. TB

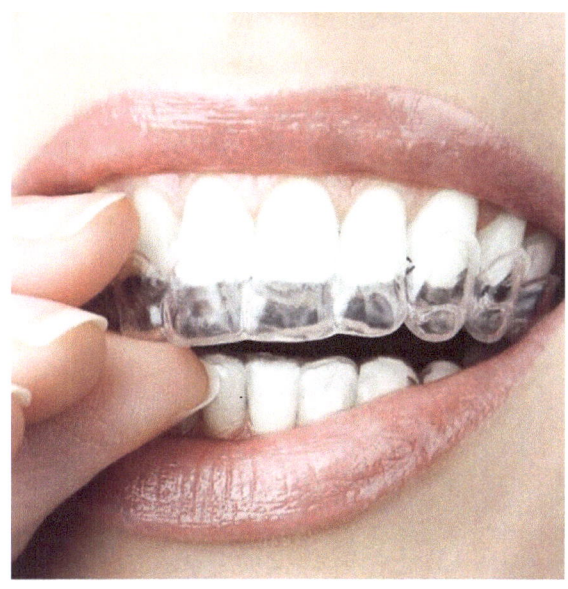

<mark>Whitening Notes</mark>

1/4/20 Took Upper and Lower Impressions with Alginate and Checked Patient shade outside with Natural Sunlight and Patient Shade is ~~A2~~ TB, A3.5, Took Before Photos

Note: Line Strike Through and Initial When Need To Correct

1/4/20 Patient came in to Try in Whitening Trays and the Fit was good, Went over Use of Whitening Gel and had Patient Sign Consent Form. Gave patient case and 4 tubes of Opalescence 20%
NV: Check Shade after Whitening Take After Photos, Composite #8 MIFL
-Dr.RK, Asst. TB

1/16/20 Checked Patient shade outside with Natural Sunlight and Went from A3.5 to A1, Patient is pleased with outcome, Placed Topical, 1 Carpule of Lidocaine 1:100, Patient did well with Anesthetic, Removed Composite restoration present and Placed Mylar stip and wedge, Placed Etch, Bond, Composite shade A1 used on I Surface and Shade A2 on Remaining surfaces to make it match Tooth #9 as Patient request. Check patient bite and check Contacts no overhangs present. Polish with Prisma Gloss. Took Post Photos, Went over P.O Instructions for Anterior Composites.
NV: Recall
-Dr.RK, Asst. TB

4/20/20 Patient called and said was moving out of state and will need records transfer to New office at Dr. Smigelski 1333 South Peters Rd, Bridget Jones 44120, Mailed Certified Mail on 4/20/20.
-TB

4/20/20 INACTIVE
-TB

Reactivate Note

6/22/27 Patient Called and wants to be Reactivated to be seen since she moved back into town and is having some Dental Issues. -TB

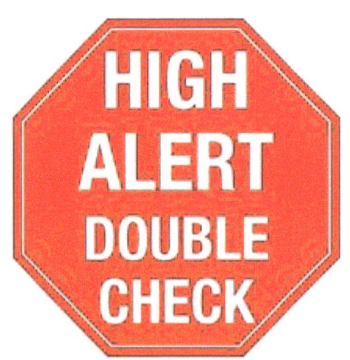

Pre-Med Note

6/27/27 New Health History Done and Patient now needs Pre-med due to Hip Replacement Per her General Physician Advised her, Pan, 4 Bw's , Soft Tissue not within normal limits and Pocket readings of 5 and above with bleeding present during probing. Comprehensive Exam Recommendations Perio and Deep Scaling but Patient Refuses and Wants Complete Dentures in placed after Remaining teeth are extracted. #3,5,12,17,24,25,29,30. Had patient sign refusal. NV: Impressions for Immediate Dentures
-Dr.RK, Asst. TB

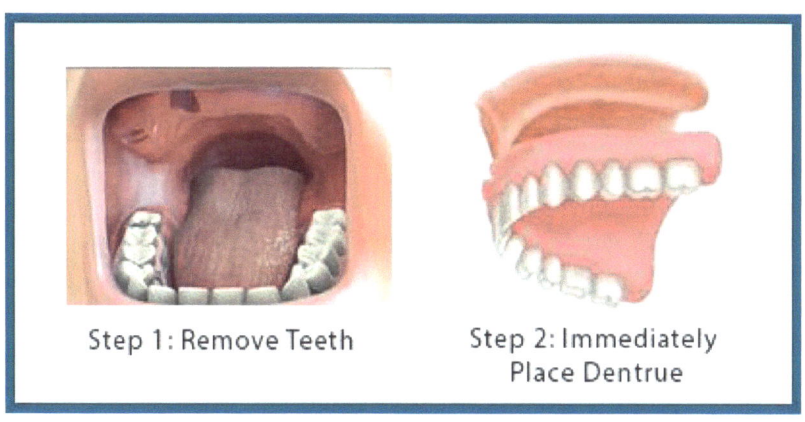

Step 1: Remove Teeth

Step 2: Immediately Place Dentrue

Immediate Denture Impressions Notes

7/1/27 Took Impressions for Immediate Dentures with Alginate sent to NDX for Custom Trays
NV: Final Impressions w/Custom Trays
-Dr.RK, Asst. TB

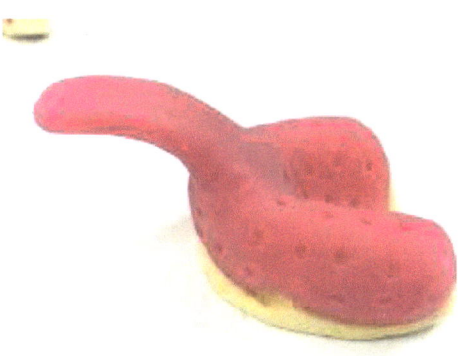

Custom Tray Notes

7/3/27 Customs Trays Tried in and Impressions Taken with Alquaseal and Bite Registration
taken with wax and Sent To NDX
NV: Wax Try-In
-Dr.RK, Asst. TB

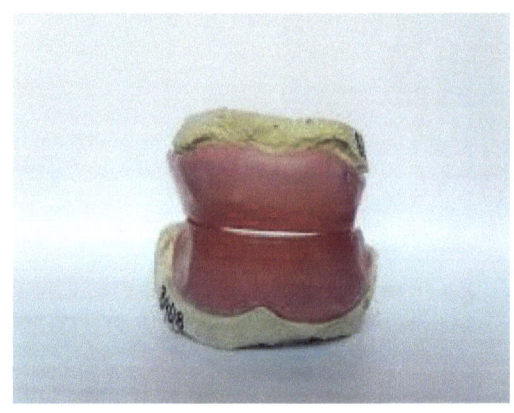

<mark>Wax Try-In Notes</mark>

7/10/27 Wax Try-in and Shade Chosen A2 along with Shape Curved chosen, Midline Indicated on Wax. Sent to NDX for Completion
NV: Extractions #3,5,12,17,24,25,29,30 and Deliver F/F
-Dr.RK, Asst. TB

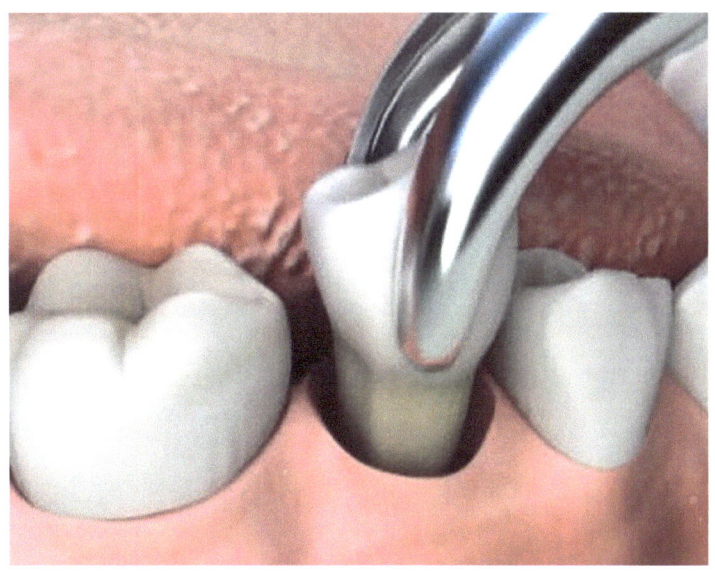

<mark>Extractions & Seat F/F Notes</mark>

7/14/27 Patient took Pre-med 1 Hour Prior, Reviewed HH, B.P 120/80, Had Patient Rinse with antiseptic Rinse Prior to seating, N20 30/40 , Placed Topical, Used 2 Carps of Lidocaine, 2 Carps of Citanest, Simple Extractions on Teeth #3,5,12,17,24,25,29,30, Removed all without complications and removed any bony fragments as well as used Saline Solutions to do final rinse of oral cavity prior to Delivering Dentures. Check patient bite as best as possible with patient being fully Anesthetized. Went over PO Instructions and RX Give For Pain Iburphope 800 mg 1 every 4 hours per pain and did not prescribe narcotics due to history, If in between dosage OTC Tylenol. Patient felt clear headed before leaving with Driver.
NV: P.O Check and Adjustments

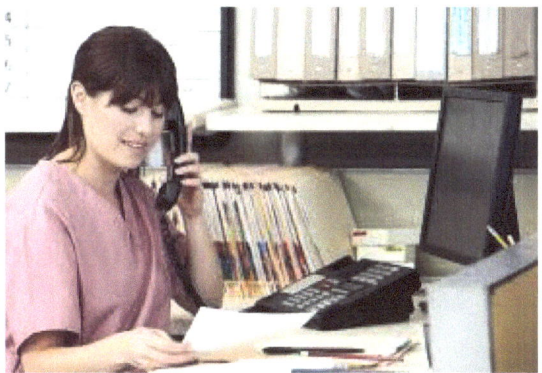

<mark>P.O Notes on Calls</mark>

7/15/27 P.O Call Patient doing well but sore and has not eaten anything, Doctor advised her to drink Ensure and to take a mult-Vitamin
-Dr.RK, Asst. TB

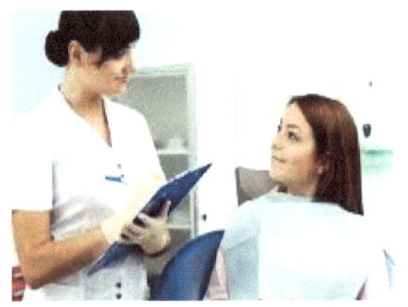

P.O Visit Notes

7/17/27 Patient is doing well with Dentures and Minor adjustments made, Tissue appears to be healing normal. Patient no longer needs Pain medicine and stopped the next day.
NV: Oral Tissue Exam & Dentures Cleaned
-Dr.RK, Asst. TB

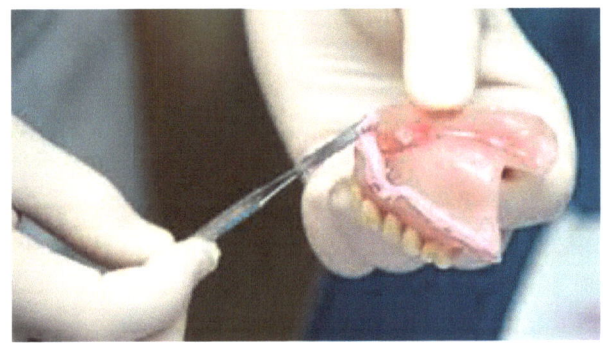

Soft Reline Notes

8/20/27 Patient came in to the office as a walk in and Maxillary Denture was loose, We did a soft Reline in office with Soft Reline X.
NV: Oral Tissue Exam and Dentures Cleaned
-Dr.RK, Asst. TB

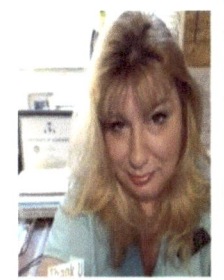

WEBSITES
STUDENTS *https://dentalindexjr.com*
DENTAL PROFESSIONALS *https://dentalindex.com*
DENTAL ADVICE *https://thedentalgeek.weebly.com*

DENTIST WEBSITES CREATOR

TUTORING SERVICE TO ALL DENTAL ASSISTANT STUDENTS/OR ENROLL FOR ONLINE OR TRAVEL TO YOU

RESUME -ORTHODONTIC ASSISTANT.- RADIOLOGY-DENTAL ASSISTANT- ADMINISTRATIVE DENTAL ASSISTANT COURSES

PORTABLE DENTAL UNIT FOR PRACTICING SUCTING
"EVERYDAY I AM SUCTIONING"

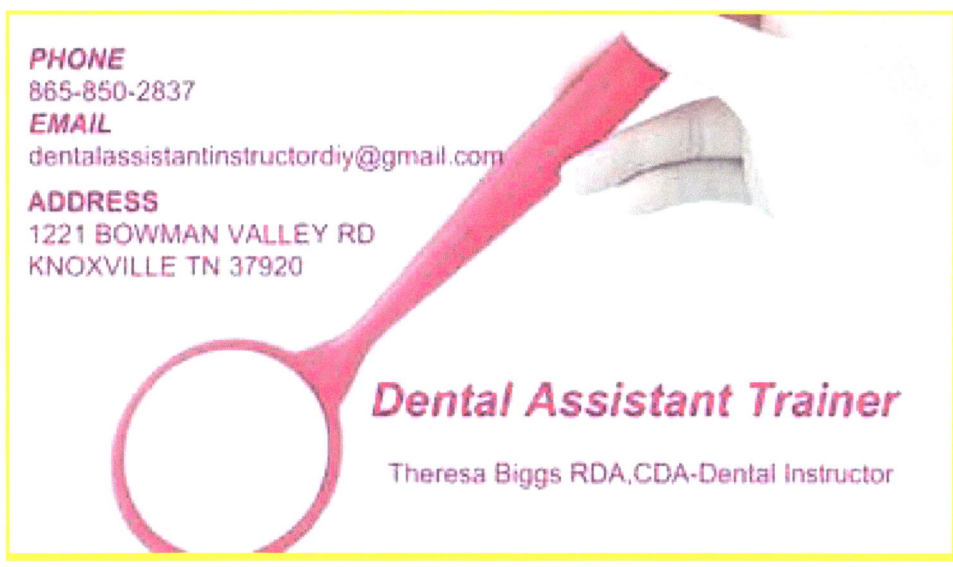

PHONE
865-850-2837
EMAIL
dentalassistantinstructordiy@gmail.com
ADDRESS
1221 BOWMAN VALLEY RD
KNOXVILLE TN 37920

Dental Assistant Trainer

Theresa Biggs RDA,CDA-Dental Instructor

Check out the Websites at
Dental Assistants and Dental Students
Help In All Dental Subjects
https://dentalindexjr.weebly.com
Or
All Dental Professionals
Dental News, Jokes, C.E
https://dentalindex.weebly.com

Want to Advertise on The Dental Geek Your Practice
Free Dental Advice Site that Refers Patients to Dentist While Traveling or In Between
Dentist

Other Books By Author
Theresa Biggs RDA, CDA
Dental Instructor

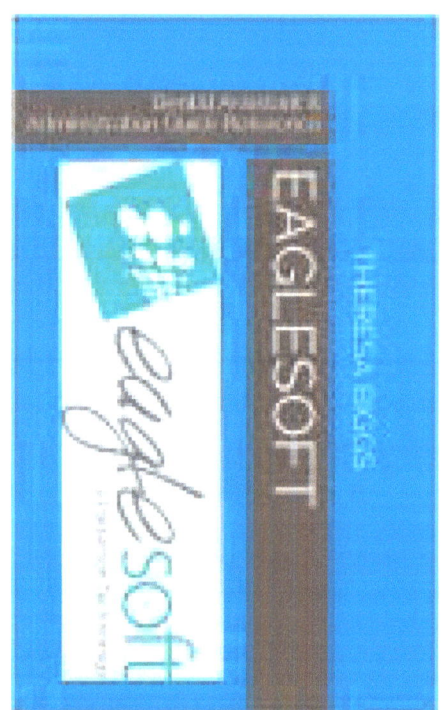

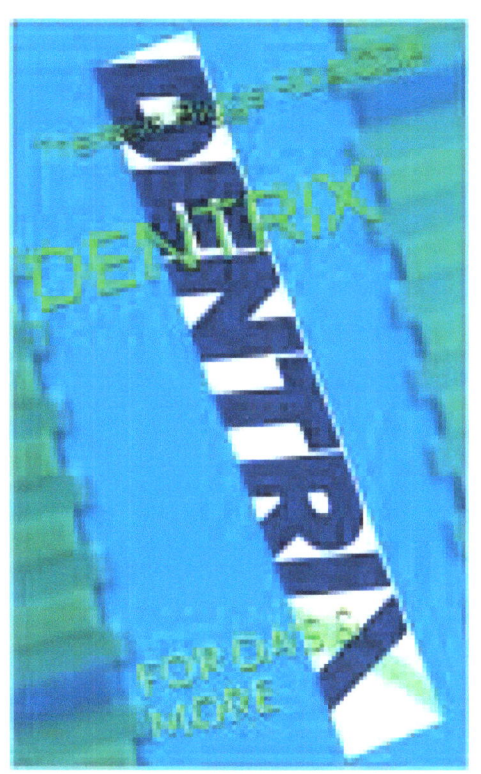

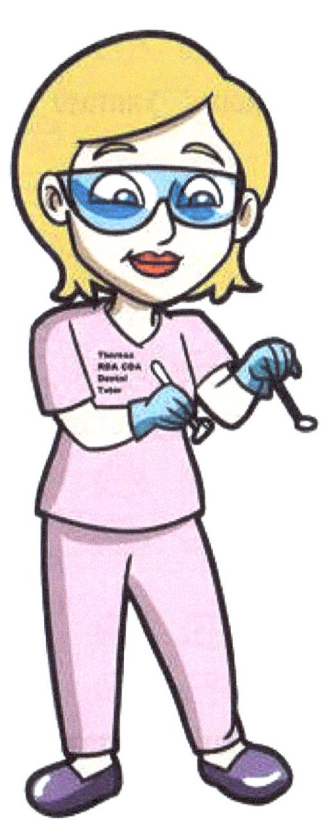

Bonus From The Dental Tutor

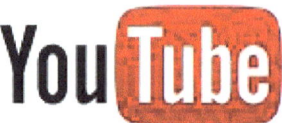

Theresa Biggs RDA CDA

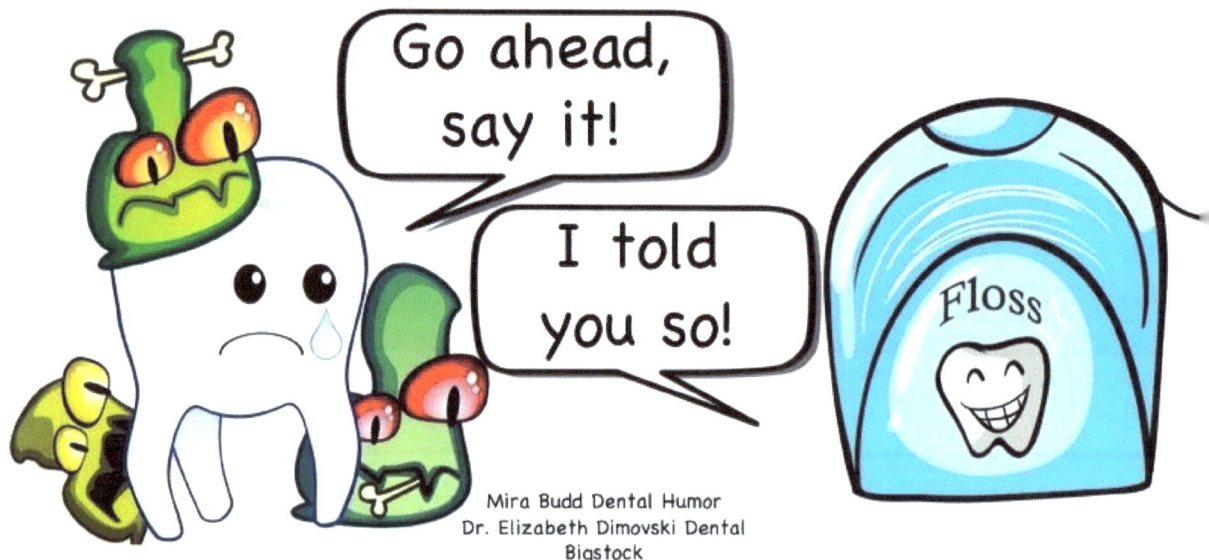

Mira Budd Dental Humor
Dr. Elizabeth Dimovski Dental
Bigstock

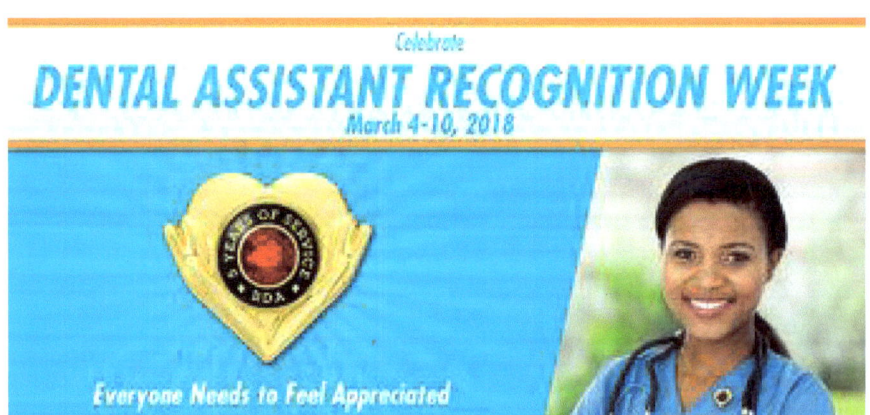

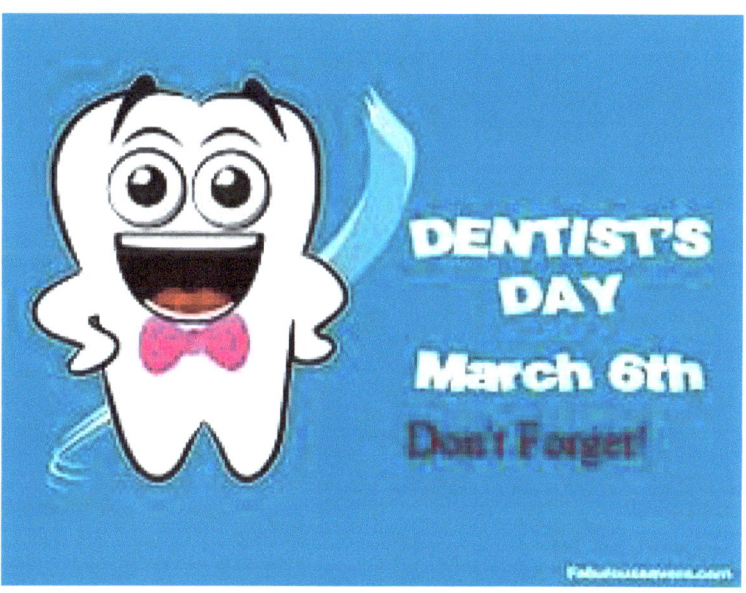

DENTIST'S DAY
March 6th
Don't Forget!

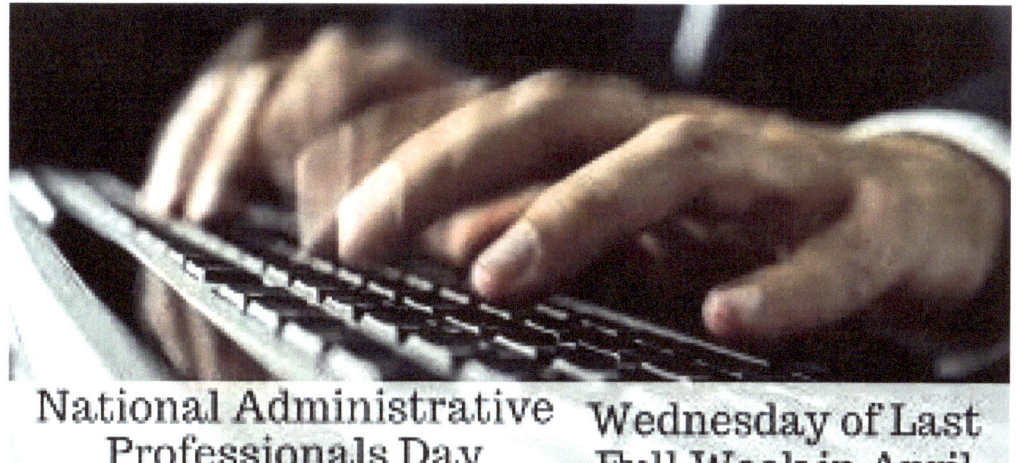

National Administrative Professionals Day
www.NationalDayCalendar.com

Wednesday of Last Full Week in April

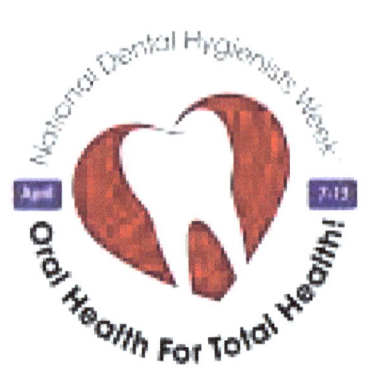

Total
Your Health Begins With Your Dental Hygienist!

National Dental Hygienists Week™
April 7- 13, 2018

Sponsored by:

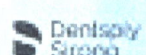 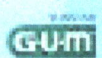

SHUT UP   - BY CARYLOLIVER

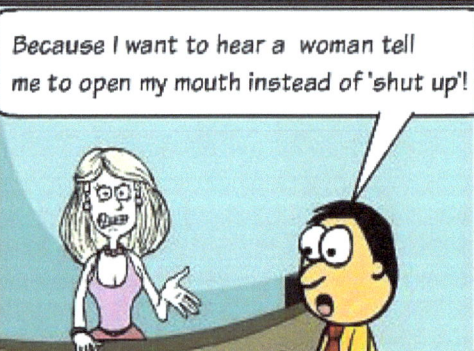

WWW.TOONDOO.COM

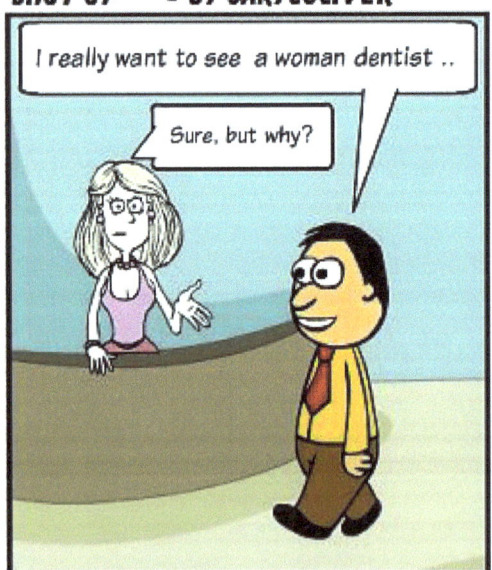

Dedication to All My Students and Family
Life is about Giving To Others

Keep On Learning

Be Kind To One Another

No I in Team!

www.ingramcontent.com/pod-product-compliance
Lightning Source LLC
Chambersburg PA
CBHW041309180526
45172CB00003B/1029